THE NEW METABOLIC CONFUSION DIET FOR SENIORS

Discover the Secrets to a Healthier and Fitter You with Delicious Recipes, Sustainable Meal Plans, and Easy Exercises for Lasting Weight Loss and Well-rounded Aging.

Vincent John Walker

DISCLAIMER

This publication is designed to provide competent and reliable information regarding the subject covered. However, the views expressed in this publication are those of the author alone, and should not be taken as expert instruction or professional advice. The reader is responsible for his or her actions. The author hereby disclaims any responsibility or liability whatsoever that is incurred from the use or application of the contents of this publication by the purchaser of the reader. The purchaser or reader is hereby responsible for his or her actions.

Table of Contents

INTRODUCTION

Introducing the "Metabolic Confusion Diet for Seniors," a comprehensive guide designed to offer you the knowledge and tools you need to rejuvenate your metabolism, enhance your well-being, and enjoy your golden years with renewed vitality. In these pages, we go on a journey that blends cutting-edge research with practical strategies, specifically created for seniors seeking to better their health and longevity.

Natural aging causes a variety of changes that have an impact on our bodies, including metabolic changes. The metabolic engine that once hummed consistently in our youth may gradually lose its efficacy, resulting in issues such as difficulty maintaining weight, fluctuating energy levels, and an increased susceptibility to chronic diseases. However, this is not the end of the story. The Metabolic Confusion Diet is an excellent way to rekindle the metabolic fire inside.

The Metabolic Confusion Diet is a complete approach that uses metabolic adaptation principles to boost your body's energy production and light your path to health. This book is your guide to navigating the diet. By cycling between precisely adjusted intervals of eating and exercise, you may wake up your metabolism, boost your energy levels, and achieve long-term advantages that outweigh the weak promises of fad diets.

Starting a transformational journey.

In the next chapters, we will delve into the heart of the Metabolic Confusion Diet, starting with an exploration of the link between aging and metabolism. Understanding the unique challenges that older people face is the foundation of the specific solutions that lay ahead. We'll clear up misconceptions regarding metabolic confusion and explain how it differs from other dietary methods by revealing the science behind it.

We invest a part of our time in preparing you mentally and emotionally since the beginning of any transformative endeavor is often the most challenging component. You'll be ready to begin your metabolic confusion journey with a clear mind and unshakable determination. Learn how to clean up your pantry and create a healthy shopping plan.

Follow these steps for long-term success:

The three distinct phases of the metabolic confusion diet are the center of this book's main topic. Phase 1 is when we jumpstart your metabolism and establish the basis for a substantial shift. Sample meals and foods will be useful references, and tips on how to exercise will help you accomplish your goals.

Phase 2 introduces variation, keeping your body on its toes and adapting. Learn how to plan your meals for maximum effect and tailor the diet to your interests and lifestyle. We'll help you stick to your training routine and coach you through more rigorous metabolic workouts that may increase your results even more.

Consolidation is critical as we approach Phase 3. This stage prepares you for a long-term lifestyle by avoiding plateaus and ensuring that your accomplishments are sustainable. We'll go over how to maintain your increased strength and how to make metabolic confusion concepts a permanent part of your lifestyle.

A comprehensive method for wellbeing

Beyond dietary considerations, we investigate lifestyle factors that work together to boost your metabolism. A comprehensive approach to well-being involves obtaining adequate sleep, managing stress, and being engaged outside of regular exercise. In addition, our meal planning and recipe section provides you with the materials you need to eat healthfully.

A Path to Empowerment

The Metabolic Confusion Diet is a journey that requires more than just physical changes. It entails approaching your senior years with zeal and confidence. Throughout this book, we encourage you to measure your progress, set acceptable goals, and celebrate each success—not only on the scale, but also in the way you feel, move, and live.

As you embark on this life-changing experience, keep in mind that age is only a number and that your health potential is limitless.

Your buddy, source of knowledge, and vehicle for empowerment is "Metabolic Confusion Diet for Seniors." Let us work together to unlock renewed vitality and create the next chapter of your active life.

AGING AND METABOLISM

The Role of Metabolism in Aging

Our bodies change as we age due to a complex and diverse process known as metabolism, which contributes to aging. The word metabolism refers to all of the chemical activity and reactions that occur inside our cells to support life. Our bodies need it to convert food into energy, build and repair tissues, and regulate a variety of physiological functions. Although metabolism is necessary for survival throughout our lives, its dynamics change as we age, which may have an impact on a variety of aspects of our health and well-being.

The following important facts illustrate the significance of metabolism in aging:

- **Energy consumption and calorie requirements:** As we age, our basal metabolic rate (BMR), which measures how much energy our bodies utilize at rest, decreases. Our bodies now need fewer calories to maintain vital functions such as breathing, circulation, and cell repair. This is referred to as a drop in BMR. If dietary choices remain the same as in prior years, the reduced calorie need may lead to weight gain.

- **Sarcopenia is the loss of lean muscle mass as we age.** Muscle tissue is more metabolically active than fat tissue, therefore it burns more calories even while at rest. As muscle mass declines, so does the body's ability to burn calories, possibly resulting in weight gain and metabolic abnormalities.

- **Metabolic Rate Variability:** While there is a general trend toward a decreased metabolic rate with age, there is significant individual diversity. A lot of factors influence how a person's metabolism changes over time, including genetics, lifestyle choices, physical activity levels, and overall health.

- **Hormonal Changes:** Hormones have an important role in metabolism. Hormone sensitivity and production may fluctuate with age. One potential impact is a decrease in the levels of many hormones, including growth hormone, thyroid hormone, and sex hormones such as estrogen and testosterone. These alterations may influence your metabolism, body composition, and overall energy balance.

- **Mitochondrial function and cellular aging:** The "powerhouses" of our cells, the mitochondria, produce energy in the form of adenosine triphosphate (ATP). Oxidative stress and accumulated damage may impair mitochondrial function over time. Reduced energy production and cellular efficiency may ensue, exacerbating age-related health issues.

- **Metabolic Stiffness:** As we age, our ability to respond to changes in food intake may decline. This metabolic stiffness may make it more difficult to metabolize different diets and increase your susceptibility to insulin resistance, a key risk factor for type 2 diabetes.

- **Inflammation and metabolism:** "Inflammation," or chronic low-grade inflammation, is associated with aging and may impact metabolism. Inflammatory activity may interfere with metabolic processes, reducing insulin sensitivity and worsening metabolic syndrome and other age-related disorders.

To promote healthy aging and treat age-related health issues, it is critical to understand the role of metabolism in aging. Age-related metabolic changes may have negative consequences, but they may be minimized by lifestyle choices such as regular exercise, a healthy diet, stress management, and enough sleep. People may endeavor to maintain their metabolic health and overall quality of life as they age by adopting a holistic approach to well-being.

Common Metabolic Changes in Seniors.

The differences that occur in the body's metabolic systems as people age are known as common metabolic changes in seniors. These changes may have an influence on many aspects of health, including energy expenditure, food intake, hormone balance, and overall well-being.

- ***A decrease in the basal metabolic rate (BMR):*** The amount of energy required by the body to keep its vital processes operating at rest is referred to as the basal metabolic rate. Their BMR tends to drop as they age. As a consequence, the body burns fewer calories when at rest, which may lead to weight gain if eating habits are not changed correctly.

- ***Reduced lean muscle mass:*** Sarcopenia, or the age-related loss of muscle mass and strength, is a major contributor to the metabolic changes that occur in the elderly. Muscle tissue consumes more calories than fat tissue due to its greater metabolic rate. When muscle mass reduces, the body's ability to burn calories decreases, which may lead to weight gain and lower metabolic efficacy.

- ***Physical Activity Decline:*** Mobility problems, chronic diseases, or lifestyle changes all contribute to a decrease in physical activity in seniors. Less physical activity may worsen muscle loss, reduce BMR, and alter metabolism.

- ***Hormonal Changes:*** Hormones have an important role in metabolism. Hormone sensitivity and production may vary with age. For example, a decrease in sex hormones (estrogen and testosterone) may affect muscle mass, bone density, and fat distribution. Additionally, a decrease in thyroid hormone levels may affect metabolic rate.

- *Insulin Sensitivity and Glucose Regulation:* As we age, we are more likely to develop insulin resistance, which impairs the body's ability to respond to insulin and manage blood glucose levels. This might lead to higher blood sugar levels, an increased risk of type 2 diabetes, and metabolic syndrome.

- *Modifications in Fat Distribution:* As individuals age, visceral fat, or fat around organs, may increase while subcutaneous fat, or fat under the skin, may decrease. This alteration increases the risk of metabolic and cardiovascular illnesses.

- *Digestive System Changes:* As people become older, their digestive systems might alter, impacting nutrition absorption and metabolism. Reduced stomach acid production and changes in gut microbiota composition might impair nutritional absorption and possibly lead to deficiencies.

- *Mitochondrial Activity:* Mitochondria, the organelles in cells that supply energy, may become less efficient and useful as they age. As a consequence, energy production may be reduced, and metabolism may decrease.

- *Chronic low-grade inflammation* and oxidative stress rise with age, influencing metabolic pathways and perhaps contributing to insulin resistance, metabolic syndrome, and other age-related diseases.

- ***Kidney function and hydration:*** As individuals age, their thirst perception and renal function decline, making dehydration more common. Proper hydration is required for metabolic processes to function normally.

- ***Drug Interactions:*** Seniors often take a variety of medications, and some of them may affect nutritional interactions and metabolism. When prescription medications for older individuals, healthcare practitioners should consider these factors.

Understanding these common metabolic changes in older adults underscores the need for a comprehensive approach to healthy aging. Regular physical activity, a balanced diet, muscle mass preservation via strength training, addressing chronic diseases, and drinking enough water may all help older people achieve optimal metabolic health.

Importance of a Balanced Diet for Healthful Aging

A balanced diet is vital for promoting healthy aging since it promotes overall well-being and reduces the effects of age-related changes. It supplies necessary nutrition, energy, and components. An individual's nutritional needs may alter as they age, making a well-balanced diet even more crucial for maintaining good health.

A balanced diet is important for healthy aging for the following reasons:

Nutrient Intake: Seniors who consume a well-balanced diet are more likely to get the essential nutrients they need, such as vitamins, minerals, proteins, carbohydrates, fats, and fiber. These vitamins and minerals are necessary for maintaining biological processes, strengthening the immune system, boosting cellular repair, and avoiding deficiencies that may lead to a variety of health issues.

Muscular Size and Strength: It's necessary to eat adequate protein to maintain muscular mass and strength, which is especially important to prevent sarcopenia (age-related muscle loss). Protein aids muscle development, repair, and overall function, allowing the elderly to remain active and self-sufficient.

Bone Health: A well-balanced diet high in calcium and vitamin D is essential for maintaining bone health and lowering the risk of osteoporosis. Adequate calcium and vitamin D consumption promotes bone density and prevents fractures, which are more prevalent in older persons.

Cardiovascular health: A well-balanced diet rich in whole grains, fiber, and heart-healthy fats (such as omega-3 fatty acids) may assist in preserving cardiovascular health. This may help to reduce the risk of heart disease, hypertension, and strokes.

Cognitive Function: Antioxidants (vitamins C and E), omega-3 fatty acids, and B vitamins have all been linked to improved cognitive health. These nutrients may support healthy brain function and contribute to a well-balanced diet, hence preventing cognitive decline.

Blood Sugar Regulate: A balanced diet high in lean proteins, fiber, and complex carbohydrates may help control blood sugar levels and reduce the chance of developing type 2 diabetes. Seniors, in particular, must maintain their blood sugar since they are more likely to develop insulin resistance.

Digestive Health: A diet rich in fiber from fruits, vegetables, whole grains, and legumes promotes regular bowel movements and reduces constipation, which is common in the elderly.

Immune System Support: A proper diet boosts the immune system's capacity to combat infections and diseases. Vitamins A, C, and E, as well as zinc and selenium, are needed for immunological function.

Managing Your Weight: A balanced diet may help seniors maintain a healthy weight. It provides the energy needed for daily activity while also avoiding excessive weight gain, which may lead to a variety of health complications.

Energy and Vitality: Consuming a variety of nutrient-dense meals provides you with the energy you need for daily chores and keeps you alert by reducing fatigue, thus boosting your overall vitality and quality of life.

Reduced Risk of Chronic Illnesses: A well-balanced diet may help lower the risk of chronic diseases including heart disease, diabetes, and certain forms of cancer, all of which grow more common as people become older.

Mental and emotional health: Omega-3 fatty acids and certain vitamins are two dietary components that have been related to better mood and mental health. A well-balanced diet may improve both emotional and cognitive wellness.

BASICS OF METABOLIC CONFUSION

What is Metabolic Confusion?

A diet and exercise approach known as metabolic confusion, sometimes known as the metabolic confusion diet or metabolic cycling, is used to boost the body's metabolism by altering the number of calories taken, the percentage of macronutrients consumed, and the quantity of activity completed. The goal of metabolic confusion is to prevent the body from growing used to a certain diet and exercise program, which may result in weight loss or fitness improvement plateaus.

The notion of metabolic confusion is based on the idea that the body adapts to predictable patterns over time. If you follow the same eating plan and exercise regimen for an extended period, your metabolism may become more efficient at processing calories and nutrients, slowing weight loss or muscle building. Metabolic confusion aims to disrupt this adaption process by introducing changes in calorie intake, nutritional ratios, and exercise intensity.

The typical mechanism of metabolic confusion is as follows:

- ***Caloric variability:*** Metabolic confusion refers to swinging between days of higher and lower caloric intake rather than consuming the same quantity of calories every day. It is thought that this variation prevents the body from growing used to a consistent energy source.

- ***Macronutrient cycles:*** Carbohydrates, proteins, and lipids may be distributed variably throughout the diet. For example, some days may focus on eating more carbohydrates, while others on eating more protein or healthy fats.

- ***Alternate-Day Fasting:*** Intermittent fasting, in which you eat and then stop eating, might cause metabolic confusion. This may encourage the body to use stored energy and regulate insulin levels.

- ***Exercise Alternative:*** Exercise for metabolic confusion requires altering the kind, intensity, and duration of the workouts. Stopping muscles from reacting, may promote continued muscular growth and fat loss.

- ***Mealtimes and Routine:*** Eating patterns may also shift, with some days focusing on fewer, larger meals and others favoring more, smaller meals. This method may prevent metabolic adaption by keeping the body guessing.

- ***People with metabolic confusion*** often choose a cyclical approach, cycling through different calorie intake, macronutrient distribution, and activity stages over preset time intervals, such as weekly or monthly cycles.

Although metabolic confusion seems promising, there is little data to support its usefulness in the scientific community. The technique is based on the concepts of metabolic adaptability and diversity in diet and exercise, but further research is needed to determine its long-term efficacy, safety, and acceptability for usage with different populations.

How Metabolic Confusion is Different from Other Diets

In contrast to prior diets, metabolic confusion adopts a unique approach to weight loss and metabolic adaption. While many diets focus on specific calorie limits, macronutrient ratios, or dietary restrictions, metabolic confusion aims to keep the body from growing used to a certain eating and exercise pattern. The following describes how metabolic confusion differs from previous diet strategies:

- *Variability and Cycling:* Metabolic confusion relies on the concept of incorporating diversity into food and exercise routines. Rather than adhering to a fixed set of guidelines, metabolic confusion entails cycling through various stages of calorie intake, macronutrient distribution, exercise intensity, and even meal time. This variety is supposed to prevent the body from plateauing and adjusting to a set regimen.

- *Avoiding Adaptation:* The purpose of metabolic confusion is to keep the body "confused" by often altering its inputs, unlike many standard diets that may produce metabolic adaptation (where the body gets more effective at using fewer calories). In theory, this helps to prevent the metabolic slowdown that might occur with chronic calorie restriction.

- ***The Cyclical Nature:*** People with metabolic disorientation often go through many phases. This might take the shape of weekly or monthly cycles, with each phase focusing on certain nutritional and exercise-related subjects. For example, one phase may focus on eating more calories and carbs, while another on consuming fewer calories and participating in more intense exercise.

- ***Exercise Accentuation:*** Traditional diets may place a high focus on calorie intake and macronutrient ratios, while metabolic confusion emphasizes exercise variation. When the kind, intensity, and duration of workouts vary, the body is less likely to adapt to a certain exercise plan.

- ***Customization:*** Metabolic confusion enables further customization depending on individual preferences and reactions. People may customize their periods of greater and lower calorie intake, macronutrient distribution, and activity intensity to their objectives and lifestyle.

- ***Long-Term Adjustment:*** Unlike diets designed for short-term results, metabolic confusion aims to give a long-term technique of weight management. Proponents of metabolic confusion argue that it may be a long-term weight loss strategy since it avoids adaptation and plateaus.

Although the concept of metabolic confusion has sparked curiosity, there has been little scientific research into its usefulness and safety compared to other dietary regimens. Individual results may vary with any diet plan, and there may be risks or problems caused by frequent adjustments in calorie intake and food distribution.

Science of Metabolic Confusion for Seniors

The "science" of metabolic confusion in seniors is based on a variety of interconnected physiological concepts and theories, however, it is important to note that this technique has not been properly studied or validated by real scientific research. The main ideas are based on how the body responds to food, physical activity, and metabolic changes. The following are some important concepts that advocates of metabolic confusion often emphasize:

- *Metabolic Adjustment*: The body is very capable of adapting to food and exercise changes. This may cause metabolic adaptation, in which the body increases its ability to utilize food and energy. This may result in a weight loss or fitness progress plateau over time.

- *Variability Disruption:* By often adjusting calorie intake, macronutrient distribution, and exercise intensity, metabolic confusion attempts to impede this adaption. According to this theory, exposing the body to fresh stimuli regularly makes adaptation more difficult.

- ***Hormonal Reaction:*** Adjusting calorie intake and macronutrient distribution may influence hormonal reactions. Changing between periods of increased and decreased carbohydrate intake, for example, may change insulin levels and other hormones that regulate metabolism and appetite.

- ***Exercise Results:*** If the kind, intensity, and duration of training programs are varied often, the body will not acquire adept in certain activities and muscle groups. This may promote the growth of lean muscle, fat loss, and overall fitness improvements.

- ***Insulin Sensitivity:*** Insulin sensitivity is thought to be influenced by a variety of metabolic factors, including intermittent fasting and carbohydrate cycling. Improving insulin sensitivity may aid with weight loss objectives and blood sugar control.

- ***Metabolic instability may influence mitochondrial adaptations.*** Supporters of this technique argue that it may improve mitochondrial efficiency and function by regularly adjusting energy demands via changes in exercise intensity and nutrient intake.

- ***Preventing Plateaus:*** The cyclical nature of metabolic confusion is intended to keep the body "guessing," to maintain a degree of metabolic difficulty that promotes continued advancement.

Even though these theories seem plausible, it is important to note that there is a lack of study on metabolic confusion, especially in senior persons. Few studies have directly examined the impact of metabolic confusion diets, particularly in older people. Instead of being backed by strong scientific facts, the bulk of the claims are based on hypothetical reasoning and anecdotal evidence.

THE BEGINNING

Measuring your total health and food

Before adopting any dietary or lifestyle changes, including the metabolic confusion diet, you should assess your existing health and nutrition. A full examination provides informative information about your starting point, identifies potential areas for growth, and aids in the construction of a personalized strategy that is aligned with your goals and medical needs. Here's how to correctly assess your current diet and health:

Medical history and current health status:

A complete physical examination will identify your starting point for wellbeing.

Nutrition Analysis:

- For a few days, keep track of your meals and fluids consumption in a food diary. Include the meal timings and quantity sizes.
- Use online tools or software to track your nutritional intake, such as calories, macronutrients (carbohydrates, proteins, and fats), vitamins, and minerals.

Body Composition

- Determine your weight and, if possible, the percentage of body fat. This may assist you in understanding your body's composition and potential areas for development.

Bloodwork:

- Consider getting blood tests to assess your blood pressure, fasting glucose, and other relevant indications.
- If necessary, talk to your doctor about tests that might reveal vitamin deficiencies.

Physical activity:

- Determine your level of physical activity right now. Keep note of the kind, frequency, and intensity of your workouts and other activities.
- Assess your aerobic fitness, strength, and flexibility.

Sleep and Stress:

- Consider your sleeping patterns and overall quality of sleep. Sleep deprivation may impair metabolism and overall health.
- Think about your stress levels and coping strategies. Chronic stress may influence health and weight management.

Dietary Preferences and Allergies.

- List any food intolerances or allergies you may have.

- Recognize your dietary requirements and preferences, as well as any cultural or ethnic limitations.

Health Goals

- Clearly define your health goals. Do you want to reduce weight, gain muscle, have more energy, improve blood sugar control, or just be healthier?

Lifestyle factors:

- Consider how your daily schedule, work, and social commitments may alter your food choices and meal times.

Mindset & Motivation:

- Consider how open you are to change. What motivates you to improve your nutrition and fitness? Are you ready to make changes?

By thoroughly examining your present diet and health, you will have a thorough understanding of your starting point and the areas where you can improve. Whether you pick the metabolic confusion technique or another nutritional strategy, this information will help you create a tailored plan that takes into account your own needs, preferences, and health goals.

Preparing mentally and emotionally.

Making long-term changes to your food and lifestyle, particularly tactics such as the metabolic confusion diet takes significant mental and emotional preparation. It requires creating the right mindset, setting acceptable expectations, and cultivating the psychological resilience needed to overcome challenges and stay committed to your goals.

- ***Establish specific goals for your health and well-being.*** Clear goals can help you remain motivated and focused, whether your goal is weight loss, greater fitness, more energy, or overall well-being.
- ***Understand Your "Why":*** Determine the reasons behind your desire to change your diet. Knowing what motivates you will provide you with a firm foundation and act as a regular reminder of the benefits you're seeking.
- ***Maintain a good attitude:*** Form an optimistic, growth-oriented mindset. Accept that change takes time and that challenges are a typical part of the journey. Place a greater focus on progress than on perfection.
- ***Manage Expectations:*** Be mindful that results may not appear immediately. Setting appropriate objectives and being patient in your efforts may help you create long-term changes.

- ***Create a Helpful Environment:*** Surround yourself with people who can assist you reach your goals. Inform your loved ones about your objectives so that they can support and keep you responsible.

- ***Develop Coping Strategies:*** Identify any hurdles or triggers that may impede your progress. Develop coping strategies for stressful circumstances, emotional eating, and temptations.

- ***Educate yourself on self-compassion:*** Be compassionate to yourself and practice it. Recognize that setbacks will occur, but instead of using them as a reason to give up, use them to learn.

- ***Recognize little victories:*** Celebrate each accomplishment, no matter how small. Celebrate your accomplishments along the road to keep yourself motivated and positive.

- ***Mindful Consumption:*** You may practice mindful eating by following your hunger signals, savoring each meal, and eating uninterrupted. Healthy eating habits foster a positive connection with food.

- ***Stay informed:*** Continue to educate yourself on food, exercise, and the basics of the metabolic confusion diet. Your commitment may be enhanced if you understand the "why" behind your choices.

- ***Manage stress*** by engaging in soothing activities such as deep breathing exercises, yoga, meditation, or hobbies.

Stress management is essential for maintaining emotional wellness.

- ***Maintain flexibility:*** Be open to changing your plan in response to your experiences. Do not be scared to make modifications if anything is not working properly.

- ***Keep Track of Your Progress:*** Record your progress using an app or a journal. Keeping a travel log allows you to assess how far you've come and identify themes that contribute to your success.

- ***Professional Guidance:*** Seek help from professionals in behavior modification and mental health, such as therapists, counselors, or registered dietitians.

The continual process of mental and emotional preparation requires self-awareness, compassion, and a commitment to your well-being. You'll be better equipped to overcome challenges, maintain consistency, and effect desired changes if you build a strong foundation of emotional and mental fortitude.

Clearing Your Pantry and Shopping List Essentials

Clearing your cupboard and making a shopping list of basics are critical stages in implementing a new nutritional strategy, such as the metabolic confusion diet. These steps assist you in creating an atmosphere that supports your health objectives while also ensuring that you have the necessary foods on hand to efficiently follow your selected plan. Here's how to empty your cupboard and make a shopping list.

Clearing your pantry:

- ***Eliminate temptations:*** Identify foods that do not fit with your new dietary objectives. This might include processed snacks, sugary meals, unhealthy oils, and high-calorie desserts. Remove these products from your pantry to avoid temptation.

- ***Check Expiry Dates:*** Go through your cupboard and remove any outdated or stale items. Maintaining fresh ingredients is critical while cooking wholesome meals.

- ***Donate or Give Away:*** If you have non-perishable products that you won't be using, consider donating them to a food bank or gifting them to friends and family who may use them.

- ***Organize:*** After eliminating unnecessary foods, reorganize your cupboard to make healthier options more accessible. Place nutritious items at eye level while keeping less healthy alternatives concealed or out of reach.

Making a shopping list of essentials

Fresh Produce:

- Mix in a variety of fruits and veggies. Choose varied hues to provide a wide spectrum of vitamins, minerals, and antioxidants.
- Leafy greens, berries, citrus fruits, cruciferous veggies, and root vegetables are all great selections.

Lean Proteins:

- Choose skinless chicken, lean cuts of meat, fish, tofu, tempeh, legumes (beans, lentils, and chickpeas), and low-fat dairy or dairy substitutes.

Whole Grains:

- Select whole grains such as brown rice, quinoa, oats, whole wheat pasta, and whole grain bread. These include complex carbs and fiber.

Healthy Fats:

- Include omega-3-rich foods like avocados, almonds, seeds, olive oil, and fatty fish (salmon, mackerel, and sardines) in your diet.

Dairy and Dairy Substitutes:

- Choose low-fat or Greek yogurt, skim milk, or dairy alternatives such as almond or soy milk.

Nuts and Seeds:

- Stock up on a variety of nuts (almonds, walnuts, pistachios) and seeds (chia seeds, flaxseeds, sunflower seeds) to add texture and nutrients to your meals.

Herbs and Spices:

- Add taste without adding calories by using herbs and spices like basil, oregano, cinnamon, turmeric, and ginger.

Condiments and Sauces:

- Use low-sodium soy sauce, vinegar, salsa, mustard, and other flavorful condiments.

Healthy Snacks:

- For filling between-meal snacks, try fresh fruit, veggie sticks with hummus, Greek yogurt, or a handful of almonds.

Hydration:

- Keep yourself hydrated throughout the day by drinking plenty of water and herbal teas.

Meal Plan Components:

- Think over the foods you'll be making and include any unique ingredients needed for your metabolic confusion meal plan.

Shopping Tip: Choose complete, unprocessed foods.

- For the best taste and nutritious content, use fresh food that is in season.
- Read food labels to make educated decisions regarding packaged goods.
- Shop the periphery of the grocery store for fresh goods, and avoid processed foods in the central aisles.

Clearing your cupboard of items that do not correspond with your objectives and developing a shopping list full of nutritional basics can help you succeed with the metabolic confusion diet or any other dietary plan you select. Remember to plan, buy wisely, and enjoy the process of providing your body with nutritious meals.

METABOLIC CONFUSION DIET PHASES

Phase 1: Jumpstart Your Metabolism

Phase 1 of the metabolic confusion diet is intended to kickstart your metabolism by implementing particular food and activity adjustments. This phase usually includes increased calorie intake, particular macronutrient ratios, and focused activities to induce a metabolic change. The objective is to inhibit adaptation, increase metabolic reactivity, and pave the way for long-term improvement. Keep in mind that the specifics of Phase 1 may vary depending on personal tastes and demands. Here's a broad overview of phase one:

Dietary Changes:

- Caloric Increase: During Phase 1, you will consume more calories than your baseline. This caloric boost is intended to offset possible metabolic adaptations from preceding calorie restriction.

- Carbohydrate Emphasis: Carbohydrates are focused in this phase to give energy and promote metabolic response. Include whole grains, fruits, veggies, and legumes in your diet.

- Protein Intake: Maintain a moderate protein intake to help preserve muscle and recover from activity. Lean protein foods such as chicken, fish, lean meats, tofu, and lentils are excellent options.

- Healthy Fats: Consume healthy fats such as avocados, nuts, seeds, and olive oil to promote satiety and general health.

- Meal Frequency: Spread out your calorie intake throughout many meals and snacks throughout the day. This helps to control blood sugar levels and avoids severe hunger.

- Hydration: Stay hydrated by drinking water throughout the day. Herbal teas and other non-calorie drinks may also be included.

Exercise Changes:

- Strength Training: Concentrate on strength training activities that target large muscular groups. This may promote muscular development and increase metabolism.

- Greater reps, lower weight: During Phase 1, you may choose higher repetitions with somewhat lower weights. This strategy may improve muscular endurance and engagement.

- Cardiovascular Exercise: Engage in cardiovascular exercises such as brisk walking, cycling, or swimming to improve overall fitness and calorie expenditure.

- Variation: To keep your body from adapting, vary your workout program regularly. This might include alternating between various workouts, intensities, and modalities.

Supplements and support:

- Nutrient support: Consider taking supplements that may help you achieve your metabolic goals, such as omega-3 fatty acids, vitamins, and minerals. However, aim to receive nutrients mostly from whole meals.

Monitoring Progress:

- Measurements: To track progress, record changes in weight, body measurements, and how your clothing fits.
- Energy Levels: Observe changes in your energy, mood, and overall well-being. Positive energy fluctuations might indicate that your metabolism is functioning properly.

MEAL PLANS AND RECIPES

Week 1: Higher Intake of Calories, with an Emphasis on Carbohydrates

Day 1:

- Breakfast: Oatmeal with berries and almonds
- Snack: Greek yogurt with honey
- Lunch: Quinoa salad with vegetables and grilled chicken
- Snack: Fresh fruit (e.g., apple or pear)
- Dinner: Baked salmon with sweet potato and steamed broccoli

Day 2:

- Breakfast: Whole grain toast with avocado and poached eggs
- Snack: Mixed nuts
- Lunch: Lentil soup with whole grain roll
- Snack: Cottage cheese with pineapple
- Dinner: Turkey stir-fry with brown rice and mixed vegetables

Day 3:

- Breakfast: Greek yogurt parfait with granola and berries
- Snack: Handful of grapes

- Lunch: Whole grain pasta with tomato sauce and lean ground beef

- Snack: Carrot sticks with hummus

- Dinner: Grilled shrimp with quinoa and roasted asparagus

Day 4:

- Breakfast: Smoothie with spinach, banana, and protein powder

- Snack: Trail mix with dried fruit

- Lunch: Chicken and vegetable wrap with whole grain tortilla

- Snack: Apple slices with peanut butter

- Dinner: Baked cod with quinoa and steamed green beans

Day 5:

- Breakfast: Whole grain pancakes with maple syrup and strawberries

- Snack: Low-fat cheese with whole-grain crackers

- Lunch: Sweet potato and black bean salad

- Snack: Orange slices

- Dinner: Beef and vegetable kebabs with brown rice

Week 2: Cardiovascular exercise and strength training are also included.

Day 1:

- Breakfast: Scrambled eggs with spinach and whole-grain toast
- Snack: Banana and a handful of almonds
- Lunch: Grilled chicken salad with mixed greens, cherry tomatoes, cucumber, and vinaigrette dressing
- Snack: Greek yogurt with a drizzle of honey
- Dinner: Baked salmon with quinoa and roasted Brussels sprouts

Day 2:

- Breakfast: Smoothie with berries, kale, Greek yogurt, and protein powder
- Snack: Orange slices and a small handful of walnuts
- Lunch: Turkey and vegetable wrap with whole grain tortilla
- Snack: Cottage cheese with pineapple chunks
- Dinner: Stir-fried tofu with broccoli, bell peppers, and brown rice

Day 3:

- Breakfast: Whole grain pancakes with sliced strawberries and a dollop of Greek yogurt
- Snack: Apple slices with almond butter

- Lunch: Quinoa bowl with black beans, corn, avocado, and salsa
- Snack: Carrot sticks with hummus
- Dinner: Grilled shrimp with sweet potato wedges and steamed asparagus

Day 4:

- Breakfast: Oatmeal with sliced banana, chia seeds, and a sprinkle of cinnamon
- Snack: Mixed nuts and dried fruit
- Lunch: Lentil soup with a whole-grain roll
- Snack: Low-fat cheese with whole-grain crackers
- Dinner: Chicken stir-fry with brown rice and assorted vegetables

Day 5:

- Breakfast: Whole grain toast with avocado, poached eggs, and cherry tomatoes
- Snack: Fresh berries and a small piece of dark chocolate
- Lunch: Whole grain pasta with tomato sauce, lean ground beef, and sautéed vegetables
- Snack: Greek yogurt parfait with granola
- Dinner: Baked cod with quinoa and roasted green beans

Day 6:

- Breakfast: Spinach and feta omelet with whole-grain toast

- Snack: Trail mix with a variety of nuts and seeds
- Lunch: Chicken and vegetable salad with mixed greens, carrots, and balsamic vinaigrette
- Snack: Sliced pear with cheese
- Dinner: Beef and vegetable kebabs with sweet potato mash

Day 7:

- Breakfast: Whole grain waffles with maple syrup and mixed berries
- Snack: Yogurt smoothie with banana and a handful of spinach
- Lunch: Quinoa salad with grilled chicken, cherry tomatoes, cucumber, and feta cheese
- Snack: Sliced peach and a small handful of pistachios
- Dinner: Shrimp and vegetable stir-fry with brown rice

Week 3: Higher Consumption of Protein

Day 1:

- Breakfast: Greek yogurt parfait with granola, mixed berries, and a sprinkle of chia seeds
- Snack: Hard-boiled eggs with a pinch of salt
- Lunch: Grilled chicken breast with quinoa and roasted vegetables
- Snack: Cottage cheese with sliced pineapple

- Dinner: Baked cod with a side of lentils and steamed broccoli

Day 2:

- Breakfast: Scrambled eggs with spinach, tomatoes, and feta cheese
- Snack: Protein smoothie with almond milk, banana, and protein powder
- Lunch: Turkey and avocado wrap with whole grain tortilla
- Snack: Handful of almonds and a piece of string cheese
- Dinner: Stir-fried tofu with brown rice and mixed vegetables

Day 3:

- Breakfast: Omelet with smoked salmon, cream cheese, and dill
- Snack: Greek yogurt with honey and a small handful of walnuts
- Lunch: Chickpea salad with tomatoes, cucumber, feta cheese, and olive oil dressing
- Snack: Sliced apple with almond butter
- Dinner: Grilled shrimp skewers with quinoa and roasted Brussels sprouts

Day 4:

- Breakfast: Protein pancakes with sliced strawberries and a dollop of Greek yogurt
- Snack: Cottage cheese with mixed berries
- Lunch: Lentil soup with a side of whole grain roll
- Snack: Trail mix with nuts and dried fruit
- Dinner: Chicken breast with sweet potato wedges and steamed asparagus

Day 5:

- Breakfast: Smoothie bowl with protein powder, banana, spinach, and a variety of berries
- Snack: Hard-boiled eggs with a sprinkle of black pepper
- Lunch: Quinoa bowl with black beans, corn, avocado, and salsa
- Snack: Greek yogurt with a drizzle of honey
- Dinner: Baked salmon with quinoa and roasted green beans

Day 6:

- Breakfast: Egg white omelet with tomatoes, spinach, and mushrooms
- Snack: Protein bar and a small piece of dark chocolate
- Lunch: Turkey and vegetable stir-fry with brown rice
- Snack: Low-fat cheese with whole-grain crackers
- Dinner: Beef and broccoli stir-fry with quinoa

Day 7:

- Breakfast: Protein smoothie with almond milk, banana, and peanut butter
- Snack: Cottage cheese with sliced peaches
- Lunch: Grilled chicken salad with mixed greens, cherry tomatoes, and a balsamic vinaigrette dressing
- Snack: Sliced pear with cheese
- Dinner: Shrimp and vegetable skewers with quinoa

Week 4: Workout Exercise Diet

Day 1:

- Pre-Workout Breakfast: Whole grain toast with avocado and poached eggs
- Post-Workout Snack: Protein smoothie with banana, spinach, and almond milk
- Lunch: Grilled chicken breast with quinoa, roasted vegetables, and a side of hummus
- Afternoon Snack: Greek yogurt with mixed berries
- Dinner: Baked cod with sweet potato mash and steamed broccoli

Day 2:

- Pre-Workout Breakfast: Oatmeal with sliced banana and a scoop of protein powder

- Post-Workout Snack: Cottage cheese with pineapple chunks
- Lunch: Turkey and vegetable wrap with whole grain tortilla
- Afternoon Snack: Mixed nuts and dried fruit
- Dinner: Stir-fried tofu with brown rice and assorted vegetables

Day 3:

- Pre-Workout Breakfast: Greek yogurt parfait with granola, mixed berries, and a drizzle of honey
- Post-Workout Snack: Protein bar and a small handful of almonds
- Lunch: Quinoa salad with grilled chicken, cherry tomatoes, cucumber, and feta cheese
- Afternoon Snack: Apple slices with almond butter
- Dinner: Grilled shrimp with quinoa and roasted Brussels sprouts

Day 4:

- Pre-Workout Breakfast: Smoothie with berries, protein powder, and almond milk
- Post-Workout Snack: Hard-boiled eggs with a pinch of salt
- Lunch: Lentil soup with a side of whole grain roll
- Afternoon Snack: Low-fat cheese with whole-grain crackers

- Dinner: Chicken stir-fry with brown rice and mixed vegetables

Day 5:

- Pre-Workout Breakfast: Whole grain pancakes with sliced strawberries and a dollop of Greek yogurt
- Post-Workout Snack: Yogurt smoothie with banana and spinach
- Lunch: Sweet potato and black bean salad
- Afternoon Snack: Sliced pear with cheese
- Dinner: Beef and vegetable kebabs with quinoa

Day 6:

- Pre-Workout Breakfast: Scrambled eggs with spinach, tomatoes, and feta cheese
- Post-Workout Snack: Protein smoothie with mango, protein powder, and coconut water
- Lunch: Chicken and vegetable stir-fry with brown rice
- Afternoon Snack: Trail mix with nuts and dried fruit
- Dinner: Baked salmon with quinoa and roasted green beans

Day 7:

- Pre-Workout Breakfast: Protein waffles with mixed berries and a drizzle of maple syrup
- Post-Workout Snack: Cottage cheese with sliced peaches

- Lunch: Quinoa bowl with black beans, corn, avocado, and salsa
- Afternoon Snack: Greek yogurt with a handful of walnuts
- Dinner: Shrimp and vegetable stir-fry with brown rice

Take into consideration the concepts of Phase 1 when you develop your meal plans. These principles include increasing your calorie intake, placing a focus on carbohydrates, and engaging in strength training activities. Your schedule and tastes may be accommodated by adjusting the portion sizes, the ingredients you choose, and the times at which you eat.

Recipes

Scrambled Eggs with Spinach and Tomatoes

Ingredients:

- 2 eggs
- Handful of baby spinach
- 1 small tomato, diced
- Salt and pepper to taste
- Olive oil or cooking spray

Instructions:

- Prepare a pan that does not stick by heating it over medium heat and adding a tiny quantity of cooking spray or olive oil (optional).

- Salt and pepper should be added to the eggs after they have been whisked in a bowl.

- As soon as the eggs have been beaten, pour them into the pan and let them cook for one minute, or until they begin to set.

- Include the baby spinach and chopped tomatoes in the mixture of eggs used.

- Utilizing a spatula, gently scramble the mixture until the eggs have reached the desired level of doneness and the spinach has contracted.

- After the eggs have been scrambled, place them on a dish and serve them with toast made with healthy grains and avocado slices.

Grilled Chicken Salad with Quinoa

Ingredients:

- 4 oz. grilled chicken breast, sliced
- Mixed greens (lettuce, spinach, arugula)
- 1/4 cup cooked quinoa
- Sliced bell peppers
- Sliced cucumbers
- Olive oil and balsamic vinegar for dressing

Instructions:

- On a dish, arrange the greens in a varied pattern.

- Slices of grilled chicken, quinoa that has been cooked, bell peppers, and cucumbers should be placed on top.

- To make a dressing, drizzle olive oil and balsamic vinegar over the salad.

- Give the salad a little toss to mix all of the ingredients.

- As a meal that is both well-balanced and healthful, you should enjoy the delectable and substantial salad.

Oatmeal with Almond Butter and Banana

Ingredients:

- 1/2 cup rolled oats

- 1 cup water or milk of choice

- 1 tablespoon almond butter

- 1 banana, sliced

- Chopped nuts (optional)

Instructions:

- It is necessary to bring the water or milk to a boil in a pot.

- The rolled oats should be stirred in, and the heat should be reduced to a simmer.

- Prepare the oats by cooking them, stirring them sometimes, until they reach the consistency that you choose (usually about 5-7 minutes).

- Place the cooked oats in a bowl and set it aside.

- If you so wish, you may garnish the oats with almond butter, sliced banana, and chopped almonds.
- Combine everything, and then take pleasure in a breakfast that is both warm and satiating.

PHASE II: INTRODUCE VARIATION

Optimizing Your Meal Structure

Structuring your meals for maximum outcomes on the metabolic confusion diet entails meticulously organizing your nutrition to support your objectives, maintain energy levels, and avoid metabolic adaption. Here's how to organize your meals for success:

Balanced Macronutrients:

- Each meal should include a good mix of carbs, proteins, and healthy fats.
- Carbohydrates provide energy, proteins aid in muscle repair and development, while healthy fats promote satiety and general well-being.

Portion Control:

- To prevent overeating, keep your portion proportions in check.
- Use visual clues such as your hand to estimate protein, carbohydrate, and fat meal amounts.

Timing of meals:

- Spread out your meals and snacks throughout the day to maintain consistent energy levels and avoid excessive hunger.
- Aim for three major meals plus one or two snacks as required.

Post-workout Nutrition:

- After an exercise, consume a balance of carbs and proteins to aid muscle repair and replace glycogen reserves.

High-quality carbohydrates:

- Concentrate on complex carbs such as whole grains, fruits, and vegetables.
- These give consistent energy and necessary nutrients.

Lean proteins:

- Choose lean protein options such as chicken, fish, lean meats, tofu, lentils, and low-fat dairy.
- Protein promotes muscle maintenance and development while also providing a sensation of fullness.

Healthy fats:

- Include healthy fats from avocados, nuts, seeds, and olive oil.
- Fats aid in hormone synthesis and make you feel full.

Fiber-rich foods:

- Include foods high in fiber, such as vegetables, fruits, whole grains, and legumes.
- Fiber aids digestion, regulates hunger, and improves gut health.

Hydration:

- Drink water all day to keep hydrated.
- Hydration is vital for good health and metabolism.

Limit added sugars:

- Reduce your consumption of sugary meals and drinks.
- Choose naturally sweet choices, such as entire fruits.

Variety:

- Aim for a diverse diet to ensure you acquire a broad spectrum of nutrients.
- Experiment with various cuisines to keep mealtime interesting.

Plan:

- Make healthy eating choices simpler by planning your meals and snacks ahead of time.
- Make meals and snacks in batches for ease.

Mindful eating:

- Eat carefully, relish each bite, and pay attention to hunger and fullness signs.

Listen to your body.

- Adjust your meal structure depending on how your body reacts. Everyone's requirements are unique.

Remember that everyone's requirements and tastes are different, so tailor your food plan to your lifestyle and goals. The idea is to provide your body with balanced, nutrient-dense meals that promote metabolic health and general well-being.

Adapting the Diet to Your Preference

Adapting the metabolic confusion diet to your tastes is critical for long-term success and durability. While the diet's primary concepts include introducing diversity, maintaining a balanced diet, and limiting metabolic adaption, there is potential for customization to meet your preferences, dietary constraints, and lifestyle. Here's how to tailor the diet to your preferences:

- Choose meals you like: Incorporate items that you enjoy while adhering to the diet's guidelines. This makes it easy to follow the strategy.
- Customize Macronutrient Ratios: Within the diet framework, modify the amounts of carbs, proteins, and fats to suit your tastes and dietary requirements.

- Culinary Creativity: Experiment with various cooking techniques, tastes, and cultures to make your meals more fascinating and pleasurable.

- Substitute Components: If you have food allergies, sensitivities, or dietary restrictions, look up appropriate alternatives for particular ingredients in the recipes.

- Meal Timing: Customize meal times to suit your schedule and tastes. To manage your metabolism, focus on consistent timing.

- Dietary Restrictions: If you follow a certain diet (e.g., vegetarian, vegan, or gluten-free), modify recipes to suit your needs.

- Portion Amounts: Adjust portion sizes based on your appetite and exercise level. If extremely tight calorie tracking does not appeal to you, avoid it.

- Intuitive Eating: Follow your body's hunger and fullness signals to drive your eating habits.

- Experiment with Stages: Try various phases of the diet to see what works best for you.

- Indulge Mindfully: Allow yourself occasional pleasures or favorite meals in moderation, and practice awareness while doing so.

- Stay Adaptable: Be willing to change your diet depending on your changing tastes, objectives, and bodily input.

- Incremental Alterations: If the diet seems overwhelming, make gradual changes to ease into the new eating habit.

Remember that the main objective is to develop a balanced and sustainable strategy that promotes your health and well-being. By personalizing the metabolic confusion diet to your tastes, you're more likely to enjoy the trip and obtain long-term outcomes that suit your specific lifestyle.

PHASE III:

CONSOLIDATION AND LONG-TERM SUCCESS

Transition to a Sustainable Eating Pattern

Transitioning to a sustainable eating pattern after the metabolic confusion diet entails striking a balance between your health objectives, dietary preferences, and long-term well-being.

- Reflect on Your Experience: Take some time to consider your experience with the metabolic confusion diet. What elements worked best for you? What did you like, and what problems did you encounter?

- Identify sustainable habits: Determine which food and lifestyle habits you find both sustainable and pleasurable. These are the habits you can adopt into your long-term diet plan.

- Focus on Whole Foods: Incorporate more whole foods into your diet. Include a mix of fruits, vegetables, lean protein, whole grains, and healthy fats.

- Listen to Your Body: Pay attention to your body's hunger and fullness signals. Eat when you are hungry, and quit when you are full.

- Choose balanced meals: Continue to prepare meals with a variety of carbs, proteins, and fats. This supports sustained energy and general wellness.

- Include meals you enjoy: Work your favorite foods into your dietary regimen. Having meals that you like contributes to a sustainable diet.

- Portion Control: Use portion control to avoid overeating. Use mindful eating strategies to enjoy your meals.

- Plan: Plan your meals and snacks ahead of time to make healthy eating easier.

- Be Flexible: Give yourself the freedom to enjoy special events and occasional delights without guilt.

- Incorporate Variety: Eat a variety of meals to ensure you acquire a diverse range of nutrients. Experiment with various dishes and cuisines.

- Gradual Adjustments: Make the transition gently and gradually. Make gradual changes over time rather than entirely altering your dietary habits.

- Monitor Your Progress: Regularly, check how you feel, your energy levels, and any changes in body composition.

- Be patient and gentle to yourself: Accept the challenge of discovering a sustainable eating pattern that suits your lifestyle and enhances your health.

Maintaining results and avoiding plateaus

Maintaining success and avoiding plateaus after following the metabolic confusion diet requires continual dedication, clever techniques, and a focus on long-lasting habits. Here's how to sustain your success and keep making great changes:

- Embrace a Healthy Lifestyle: Change your thinking from a temporary diet to a lifetime dedication to health. Focus on developing long-term lifestyle improvements.

- Continuously Vary Your Program: Incorporate variety into your training routine. Change your training routine, intensity, and activity kinds regularly.

- Caloric Intake: As your body changes, you should modify your caloric intake to meet your energy requirements. If necessary, get advice from a qualified specialist.

- Incremental Changes: Make gradual changes to your food and exercise regimen to prevent abrupt changes that might result in plateaus.

- Mindful Eating: Practice mindful eating to become aware of your body's hunger and fullness signals. Avoid overeating and undereating.

- Strength Training: Continue to do strength training to preserve muscle mass, enhance metabolism, and promote bone health.

- Set New Goals: Set new exercise and health objectives to keep yourself motivated and involved throughout your journey.

- Monitor Progress: Evaluate your progress regularly using measurements, body composition analysis, and performance improvements.

- Stay Hydrated: Drink enough water to assist your metabolism, digestion, and general health.

- Prioritize Sleep: Get enough sleep to help you recuperate, have more energy, and maintain hormonal balance.

- Celebrate non-scale successes: Concentrate on non-scale victories like increased strength, endurance, and general well-being.

- Intuitive Eating: Listen to your body's messages and eat based on physical hunger rather than emotional impulses.

- Consistency is key: To sustain results, stick to your selected eating pattern and exercise plan regularly.

- Regular Check-Ins: Reassess your objectives, habits, and progress to ensure you're on track.

- Adjust When Necessary: If you feel your progress stalling, try making strategic changes to your routine, such as your diet or exercise.

- Maintain a good attitude and concentrate on the advantages of a healthy lifestyle that extends beyond physical beauty.

TAILORING THE DIET TO YOUR NEEDS

Adapting Metabolic Confusion to Dietary Restrictions

Adapting the metabolic confusion method to dietary limits demands careful preparation and innovation to ensure you achieve your nutritional requirements while adhering to the diet's principles. Here's how to adapt the metabolic confusion diet to meet typical food restrictions:

Vegetarian or vegan?

- Plant-based protein sources include beans, lentils, chickpeas, tofu, tempeh, seitan, quinoa, nuts, and seeds.

- Omega-3s: Include plant-based omega-3 fatty acid sources such as flaxseeds, chia seeds, walnuts, and algal supplements.

- B12 and Iron: Keep track of your vitamin B12 and iron consumption, since vegetarian or vegan diets frequently have lower levels of these elements. Consider fortified meals or supplements if required.

Gluten-Free:

- Grains: Choose gluten-free whole grains such as rice, quinoa, millet, and certified gluten-free oatmeal.

- Flour: For cooking and baking, use gluten-free flour such as almond flour, coconut flour, and chickpea flour.

- Read labels carefully to avoid gluten-containing ingredients in packaged meals.

Dairy-Free:

- Calcium: To maintain appropriate calcium intake, consume fortified dairy-free milk substitutes such as almond milk, soy milk, or oat milk.

- Non-Dairy Yogurt: Select yogurt made from coconut, almond, soy, or cashew.

- Avocados, almonds, seeds, and olive oil are all excellent sources of healthful fats.

Nut and Seed Allergies:

- Protein options that are not nuts or seeds include lean meats, poultry, fish, dairy (if not allergic), legumes, and gluten-free grains.

- Healthy Fats: Consume healthy fats like avocados, olive oil, and coconut oil.

Specific allergies or sensitivities:

- Substitutions: Determine appropriate substitutions for allergic items in recipes. If you are sensitive to peanuts or almonds, you may use sunflower seed butter instead.

- Consult a Professional: Work with a dietician to verify that you are obtaining all of the necessary nutrients despite your dietary limitations.

Medical Conditions (for example, diabetes, high blood pressure):

- Carbohydrates: To control blood sugar levels, monitor your carbohydrate consumption and pick complex carbohydrates.
- To regulate blood pressure, choose low-sodium alternatives and restrict your intake of processed meals.

Other dietary restrictions:

- Research and Planning: Look for recipes and resources that are tailored to your dietary demands and constraints.
- Experiment with different cuisines and cooking ways to broaden your possibilities.

Strategies for Overcoming Challenges

Overcoming hurdles when following the metabolic confusion diet, or any other dietary plan, is critical to long-term success. Here are some ideas for overcoming typical problems and staying on track:

Cravings and temptations:

- Prepare for occasional delights and savor them wisely.
- Keep healthy options on hand in case cravings occur.
- Use portion control to fulfill urges without jeopardizing development.

Social Events and Dining Out:

- Check the menu ahead of time and choose healthier options.

- Eat a well-balanced supper or snack before attending an event to prevent overindulgence.

- Choose grilled, baked, or steamed alternatives, then ask for sauces or dressings on the side.

Time constraints:

- Preparing meals and snacks ahead of time ensures that healthy alternatives are accessible.

- Choose fast and simple recipes, or utilize food delivery services.

Boredom or lack of motivation:

- To keep things fresh, change up your eating plan and workout program.

- Setting fresh objectives and tracking your progress can help you remain motivated.

Plateaus:

- To break past plateaus, adjust your calorie intake and workout program.

- Vary your training intensity, kind, and duration.

Emotional eating:

- Practice mindfulness and become aware of your emotional eating triggers.
- Find non-food strategies to deal with your emotions, such as taking a walk or practicing deep breathing.

Lack of support:

- Communicate your aspirations to friends and family, requesting their understanding and support.
- Seek out online networks or support groups dedicated to your eating strategy.

Traveling:

- Pack healthy snacks and make healthful choices while on the run.
- To make healthier choices, research the eateries and food shops near your location.

Stress:

- Practice stress-reduction strategies such as meditation, yoga, and deep breathing.
- Prioritize self-care to reduce stress.

Lack of Time to Exercise:

- Include brief periods of activity throughout the day, such as walking or bodyweight exercises.
- Choose effective exercises, like as HIIT, that deliver maximum results in a short period.

Plate Preparation and Cooking Skills:

- Invest time in mastering basic culinary methods and progressively improve your talents.
- Learn about meal prep ideas to save time throughout the week.

Financial constraints:

- Choose cheap, nutrient-dense foods such as beans, lentils, whole grains, and seasonal vegetables.
- Buy in bulk whenever feasible to save money.

Fear of Failure:

- Accept setbacks as learning opportunities, rather than failures.
- Set reasonable objectives and recognize little accomplishments along the way.

LIFESTYLE FACTORS FOR IMPROVED METABOLISM

The Importance of Sleep for Metabolism

Sleep regulates a variety of physiological systems, including metabolism. Getting enough good sleep is critical for keeping a healthy metabolism and general well-being.

Energy Regulation:

- Sleep regulates the balance between energy intake (calories ingested) and energy expenditure (calories burned).
- A lack of sleep may upset this equilibrium, resulting in overeating and weight gain.

Hormonal Balance:

- Sleep impacts the release of hormones that regulate metabolism, such as insulin, cortisol, and leptin.
- Disrupted sleep patterns may cause insulin resistance, elevated cortisol (a stress hormone), and impaired hunger management.

Appetite Regulation:

- Sleep deprivation may cause abnormalities in the hormones ghrelin and leptin, which control appetite and fullness.

- Overeating is commonly caused by a lack of sleep, which increases ghrelin (an appetite-stimulating hormone) and decreases leptin (a satiety hormone).

Muscle Recovery and Growth:

- Sleep is necessary for muscle repair and development, which are required to sustain a higher metabolic rate.
- Deep sleep causes the production of growth hormone, which promotes muscular development.

Restore Cellular Function:

- Sleep enables cells to repair and rejuvenate, hence ensuring appropriate metabolic function.
- During sleep, the body repairs and heals tissues, which helps with overall metabolic health.

Thermoregulation:

- Sleep regulates body temperature, which is related to metabolic rate.
- Poor sleep may impair temperature control and perhaps affect metabolism.

Circadian rhythms:

- Adequate sleep is required to maintain a healthy circadian rhythm, which regulates the timing of metabolic activities.

- Circadian rhythm disruptions, such as inconsistent sleep patterns, have been shown to alter metabolism.

Fat Metabolism:

- Sleep helps regulate the body's usage of fat for energy.
- Sleep deprivation may impede fat metabolism and storage, resulting in weight gain.

Overall health:

- Chronic sleep deprivation increases the risk of obesity, type 2 diabetes, cardiovascular disease, and other metabolic disorders.

Stress Reduction:

- Adequate sleep reduces stress levels, which may lead to a healthy metabolism and less inflammation.

Brain health:

- Sleep is necessary for cognitive function and decision-making, which may influence eating preferences and lifestyle habits.

Recovery after Exercise:

- Sleep is essential for post-workout recovery since it allows the body to rebuild muscle tissue and restore energy reserves.

Prioritizing sleep is critical for keeping a healthy metabolism and overall wellbeing. Aim for 7-9 hours of quality sleep every night, have a consistent sleep schedule, develop a soothing bedtime ritual, and create a sleep-friendly atmosphere to support your metabolic health.

Managing Stress and its Effect on Aging

Stress management is critical to fostering good aging and general well-being. Chronic stress may have a major influence on a variety of physiological systems, including the aging process.

Effects of Stress on Aging:

- Cellular Aging: Chronic stress may accelerate cellular aging by shortening telomeres, which are protective caps at the ends of chromosomes. Telomere shortening has been linked to several age-related disorders.

- Inflammation: Stress causes inflammation, which has been linked to several age-related disorders, including cardiovascular disease, diabetes, and cognitive decline.

- Prolonged stress may alter hormonal equilibrium, resulting in elevated cortisol levels. Elevated cortisol levels are linked to poor health and may exacerbate metabolic problems.

- Cognitive Decline: Chronic stress may lead to cognitive decline and memory issues over time.

- Immune System: Stress reduces the immune system's reaction, rendering people more vulnerable to infections and diseases.

Strategies for Managing Stress:

Practice awareness and meditation.

Mindfulness and meditation practices may help you decrease stress and relax.

These techniques enhance emotional control and resistance to shocks.

a. Regular exercise helps to produce endorphins, which are natural mood enhancers that counteract stress.

b. Engage in activities you like, such as walking, yoga, swimming, or dancing.

c. A healthy diet includes fruits, vegetables, whole grains, lean meats, and healthy fats.

d. Nutrient-dense diets improve the body's stress response and general wellness.

e. Adequate Sleep: Prioritize quality sleep to reduce stress and improve general well-being.

   - Aim to get 7-9 hours of sleep per night.

f. Time Management: Use your time wisely to prevent feeling overwhelmed.

g. Break down projects into smaller chunks and prioritize them.

h. Deep breathing exercises might help you relax and decrease tension.

i. Limit your coffee and alcohol intake: Too much caffeine and alcohol may increase stress and alter sleep patterns.

j. Engage in Pastimes: Find hobbies that you like to distract your attention away from tension and encourage relaxation.

k. Mind-Body Practices: Try exercises like tai chi, qigong, or progressive muscle relaxation to enhance calm and the mind-body connection.

l. Limit media exposure: Set limits on media intake, especially news that might cause stress.

m. Practice Thanks: Every day, reflect on the good things in your life and express gratitude.

Managing stress correctly is critical for supporting good aging and sustaining overall health. By using stress management practices and living a balanced lifestyle, you may reduce the harmful impacts of stress and improve your well-being as you age.

TRACKING PROGRESS AND ADJUSTMENTS

Setting realistic goals for health and wellness.

Setting realistic health and wellness goals is critical for bringing about long-term change and success. Unrealistic objectives may cause frustration and despair, but attainable goals can bring drive and a feeling of success. How to Set Realistic Goals:

a. Be Specific: Define what you intend to accomplish. Avoid ambiguous objectives like "become healthy" and instead identify activities like "exercise three times per week."

b. Break down bigger goals: If you have a huge objective, divide it into smaller, more manageable tasks. This makes the procedure easier and less intimidating.

c. Make them measurable: Set objectives that can be monitored and assessed. This enables you to assess your progress and make any required modifications.

d. Set Attainable Objectives: Select goals that are tough but yet achievable. Setting too ambitious objectives might cause burnout.

e. Set both short-term and long-term objectives for a balanced approach.

f. Use the SMART criterion, which stands for specific, measurable, attainable, relevant, and time-bound. Applying these criteria ensures that your objectives are well-defined and attainable.

g. Focus on Behavior, Not Results: Prioritize actions and behaviors above outcomes over which you have no direct influence. Consider eating more veggies rather than reducing a set amount of weight.

h. Consider Your Lifestyle: Make sure your objectives align with your everyday life and activities. A realistic objective should be something you can regularly achieve.

i. Set Process and End Objectives: Combine process goals (your activities) with outcome goals (results you want). This offers a well-rounded perspective.

j. Celebrate Minor Wins: Recognize your accomplishments along the road, even if they are small steps toward your overall objective.

k. Reevaluate and Adjust: Reassess your objectives regularly to verify they are still relevant, and make any necessary adjustments.

l. Be patient: Understand that development takes time. Be patient and consistent in your efforts.

m. Focus on Health, Not Perfection: Instead of perfection or a certain look, strive for improvement and improved health.

n. Be adaptable: life is unexpected. Be willing to alter your aims in response to changing circumstances.

Setting realistic health and wellness objectives allows you to build a plan for implementing the changes you want. Breaking down your objectives, measuring your progress, and making modifications as required increases your chances of long-term success in enhancing your well-being.

Identifying plateaus and implementing necessary changes

Plateaus are prevalent in health and wellness journeys when progress seems to stagnate despite your efforts. Identifying plateaus and making required modifications is critical to maintaining progress toward your objectives.

a. Monitor Progress: Keep track of your progress regularly using measurements, pictures, fitness benchmarks, and your general mood.

b. Identify Patterns: Look for patterns in your development. If you find a continuous lack of progress over many weeks, you may be at a plateau.

c. Nutrition: Reassess your eating habits. Are you continuously adhering to your preferred eating pattern? Are the portion sizes accurate?

d. Review your exercise regimen. Have you been doing the same workouts at the same intensity for a lengthy period?

e. Check Sleep and Stress: Assess your sleep quality and stress levels. Inadequate sleep and prolonged stress might impede growth.

f. Change Intensity: Step up the intensity of your exercises. Increase the weight you lift, experiment with interval training, or lengthen your workouts.

g. Introduce fresh workouts to test various muscle areas while preventing adaption.

h. Modify Reps and Sets: Change the amount of repetitions and sets in resistance exercises to stress your muscles differently.

i. Alter the length, intensity, and kind of cardio exercises to prevent reaching a plateau.

j. Nutritional Adjustments: If your progress has halted, try altering your calorie intake or macronutrient ratios to meet your objectives.

k. Try a Rest Week: Schedule a week of lower-intensity exercises to enable your body to recuperate and reset.

l. Change the Regimen: Try a new fitness class or activity to completely change your training routine.

m. Review Nutritional Quality: Make sure your food is balanced and nutrient-dense. Concentrate on healthy meals and minimize processed stuff.

n. Avoid Overtraining: Make sure you provide enough time for recuperation. Overtraining may cause plateaus, even regression.

o. Be patient: plateaus are a regular part of the process. Stay patient and devoted to your objectives.

p. Celebrate Non-Scale Victories: Look beyond the numbers on the scale and recognize other accomplishments such as increased strength or energy.

LONG-TERM MAINTENANCE AND BEYOND

Transition to a Sustainable Dietary Pattern

Transitioning to a sustainable dietary pattern is a long-term strategy that focuses on developing a balanced and pleasurable style of eating that you can stick with over time. Here's how to ensure a seamless transition:

a. Reflect on Your Objectives: Think about your health goals, preferences, and values. These features should be reflected in your new eating pattern.

b. Gradual Changes: Avoid abrupt transitions. Make minor, incremental modifications to your dietary habits over time.

c. Prioritize Entire Foods: Focus on whole, minimally processed foods such as fruits, vegetables, lean meats, whole grains, and healthy fats.

d. Create balanced meals that contain a variety of carbs, proteins, and fats to meet your energy requirements.

e. Mindful Eating: Pay attention to hunger and fullness signs. Eat leisurely and enjoy your food.

f. Hydration: Drink enough water throughout the day to help your digestion and general health.

g. Portion Control: Use portion control to prevent overeating. Pay attention to your body's cues of fullness.

h. Allow yourself occasional pleasures or meals that you like, but do it consciously and in moderation.

i. Meal Planning: Make healthy eating and snacking easier by planning ahead of time.

j. Diversity and Variety: Eat a variety of meals to ensure you obtain a broad range of nutrients. Experiment with various dishes and cuisines.

k. Listen to Your Body: Notice how various meals make you feel. Adjust your diet according to how your body reacts.

l. Learn Culinary Skills: Improve your cooking abilities to prepare tasty and healthy meals at home.

m. Reduce your consumption of sugary and highly processed meals gradually.

n. Focus on Fiber: To aid digestion and satiety, consume fiber-rich meals such as whole grains, fruits, vegetables, and legumes.

o. Check-Ins: Check in regularly to see how you're feeling, how much energy you have, and any changes in your body.

p. Celebrate Progress: Recognize your accomplishments, whether they are tiny changes in your eating habits or big health milestones.

CONCLUSION

To summarize, the road toward better health, well-being, and long-term vitality is a dynamic and diverse activity. Throughout our investigation of the "Metabolic Confusion Diet for Seniors" and associated issues, we've looked at the complex interaction of metabolism, aging, diet, exercise, stress management, and lifestyle choices. By combining this information, we may develop a comprehensive viewpoint that will enable us to make educated choices about our long-term health.

We've discovered that metabolism, the complicated engine that drives our bodies, alters as we age. Genes, lifestyle, and hormone alterations all have an impact on these changes. The "Metabolic Confusion Diet for Seniors" is a strategic strategy that uses variations in exercise and diet to accelerate metabolism and promote healthy aging. By adopting this strategy, elders may harness the power of metabolic confusion to improve their health and maintain a healthy lifestyle.

Crucially, a balanced diet rich in nutrient-dense foods, portion management, and mindful eating are the foundations of this nutritional approach. By giving our bodies the correct fuel, we can maintain energy levels, support metabolic function, and promote healthy aging. Furthermore, consistent exercise regimens that include aerobic, weight training, and flexibility exercises are essential for preserving muscle mass, bone density, and general vitality.

However, this path entails more than simply nutrition and exercise; it also includes stress management, prioritizing sleep, and establishing a happy mentality. We've looked at how stress affects aging and how stress-reduction measures may help us feel better in general. Adequate sleep, a key component of a healthy lifestyle, regulates metabolism, cognitive function, and emotional equilibrium.

Transitioning to a sustainable dietary pattern entails establishing realistic objectives, appreciating variety in food choices, and incorporating metabolic confusion concepts into our everyday lives. By progressively applying these ideas, we may develop a lifestyle that meets our requirements, interests, and aspirations.

Finally, our road to health and well-being is a lifetime activity that needs patience, self-compassion, and a dedication to ongoing learning and improvement. The information and tactics we've discussed provide a road map for navigating the complexity of aging and metabolism, allowing us to make educated decisions that promote health, longevity, and a higher quality of life.

As we go ahead, let us remember that our bodies are extraordinary vessels capable of adaptation and change. By adopting and incorporating the ideas of the "Metabolic Confusion Diet for Seniors" into our journeys, we start on a road of empowerment, resilience, and well-being that celebrates the gift of a healthy and meaningful life.